I0429557

Legal & Disclaimer

Contents

Introduction

Do you often find yourself at some point during the day suffering from severe headaches or migraines? Perhaps you try to wing it and get your coffee or soda fix hoping it will simply go away. Or maybe at times, you take some over the counter pain medication and you do get rid of the headache, but now you find yourself drowsy and need a nap. But, as a young working adult, you don't have time for a nap, you have to do to keep going. At times you may feel like you just can't win! You have to keep going, as your day is certainly not over. Just thinking about picking up your youngest from day care after an hour of driving through downtown, before rushing to your teenager's soccer practice is enough to give you serious headaches.

We are glad to tell you that there is a better alternative. It is possible to treat headaches and migraines with natural methods, and in this book we will introduce you to the most popular essentials oils that can be used to do so. That's right, in this guide, you will learn how to make these wonderful essential oils to treat many minor illnesses, including these annoying and sometimes debilitating headaches. You will no longer be tasked with trying to wing it, or with trying to function while feeling drowsy in the middle of the day because of any over the counter or even prescription medication. Aromatherapy or use of essential oils for treatments is a wonderful option to help you feel better, and avoid any type of dependency or side effects. We will introduce you to the many benefits of adopting essential oils to ease your pain and make your life much more peaceful.

Learn in this book how to mix well the essentials oils in order to help you take care of these harmful headaches. Find out how you can maximize the effectiveness of these oils, and even if you eventually decide you do not want to prepare these oils yourself, you will learn what to look for when it's time to purchase them. We also want to ensure that you utilize these essential oils safely and that you enjoy many of their wonderful properties.

A headache can at times can transform into a migraine. If you are experiencing the following symptoms, you are most likely suffering form a migraine: severe throbbing pain encompassing your entire head, or shifting from one side to another. You will also often be very sensitive to noise, light, or smells and you may even experience blurry vision. Whatever your symptoms, sit back and relax and get ready to learn the techniques to ease the pain of these migraines and headaches with natural essential oils.

Grab Free Books Here

From time to time, I would highlight to my readers some interesting books which I found on Kindle. Subscribe to our newsletter to receive free bestselling kindle books recommendation delivered to your inbox daily. You can subscribe to our newsletter by clicking on the link below:

http://giveaway.kindleheaven.com/index.php/kindle-free-book/

It is 100% free and there will not be a single spam email. Just pure sharing of good books with my readers.

Please also like our facebook page below to get recommendation on good books to read for the day.

https://www.facebook.com/Kindle-Heaven-1651266215134798

Follow us on Twitter to get tweets on worthwhile books

https://twitter.com/KindleHeaven

Chapter 1: Benefits from Using Essential Oils

We are constantly bombarded with reminders about changing our eating habits in order to be healthier. Of course, what you eat makes a big difference in the way you feel and can help prevent many diseases and ailments, not the least of which is headaches. This is all very well and good, but since you try to eat better and control what goes into your body, doesn't it make sense to also try to medicate better? Let's talk in detail of the many benefits associated with the use of essentials oils.

Essential oils vs prescription drugs

As you have probably already noticed, when you are prescribed a drug, you are urged to read an extensive list of possible side effects. The same cannot be said of essential oils.

When your body has to deal with an unknown, synthetic substance contained in prescription drugs, it struggles with what to do with that foreign substance. Yes, it can treat some of your health conditions, but some traces of the medication can remain in your body for long periods of time before it is fully eliminated. Quite to the contrary, natural plants, herbs and oils, can be easily metabolized by your system. When an essential oil is done treating the needed area of your body, it will then move to the liver and kidneys and be naturally eliminated.

Another big difference is that drugs toxify your body while oils can work to detoxify it. Have you ever heard that if you take too many antibiotics, your immune system will become weaker and incapable to fighting off infections on its own? This is what happens, because the bacteria, both good and bad, will be destroyed by antibiotics, as opposed to essential oils, which only eliminate the bad and leave the good alone.

Although prescription drugs can relieve the pain of headaches and migraines, they can also at times disturb some of your other body functions—this is commonly referred to as side effects—and they can also cause light to extreme drowsiness. Oils actively work at restoring your natural bodily functions, so there are generally no side effects to be worried about when taking them.

Many health benefits

Because of their multiple properties, essentials oils can help you physically, mentally, and even emotionally. They are used to help with may medical conditions, including but not limited to: headaches, migraines, digestive problems, mood disorders, sleep disorders, skin conditions, allergies, bug bites, cuts, burns, boosting immune system and energy levels, weight loss, muscular and joint pain, and slowing the process of aging.

Don't be afraid to use essential oils, they are not synonymous with fat or fatty acids. The oils are primarily composed of plant extracts, and it does take a large amount of the plants and herbs to get a tiny quantity of oil. In general essential oils should not be applied directly to your skin, and with a few exceptions, are usually not made for oral consumption. Of course and as always, if you have questions regarding the safety or use of oils, you should discuss with your primary care physician. If you are taking prescription drugs, you also want to verify with a health professional that there is no danger of negative interactions to taking the essential oils as well. It's possible by speaking with your doctor, you could even eventually come up with a plan to eliminate some of your pharmaceutical medications and replace them with natural options, such as essential oils.

Cost effective

If you think about it, when you are sick, even if you are only battling a cold, going to the doctor can end up costing you a lot of money. You will have to come up with a minimal copay for the visit, and that's if you are able to get an appointment with and go to your regular doctor and not a walk in clinic or an emergency room, where the copay is much higher (let's assume you will pay in average $30). Generally, depending on what is found, you will be prescribed some medications, and again you will have to come up with an additional $10 or more of copay. Let's say you need to follow up with the doctor, add another $30 co-pay. These amounts are of course assuming you have medical insurance, and obviously if you do not they would be much higher.

Comparatively speaking, A few drops of essential oils should not cost you more than a few dollars at the most. You also don't have to drive to the doctor or the pharmacy, saving some additional gas money and precious time. The fact that essential oils are much cheaper than prescription drugs is certainly another benefit or advantage to consider.

Essential oils properties

Because there are so many different oils, made with a variety of herbs and plants, the properties are unlimited. As mentioned above, they can help treat a myriad of health conditions. Oils can be combined for more efficiency or can be used on their own. If you have a problem, you can be certain that there is a natural solution out there that you can try to improve it. It should be noted that there is no certainty that essential oils can cure diseases, but they can absolutely help relieve certain symptoms, and provide an overall improved well-being.

Aromatherapy is in fact a therapy, or alternative medicine, that can provide this very type of relief. By utilizing a blend of essential oils, aroma therapists can apply the oils, suggest the inhalation of the oils, and/or even utilize water immersion to create the desired effect.

Chapter 2: Two Methods To Prepare Essential Oils

Now that you are convinced that essential oils are a good investment of your time and minimal expenses, it's time to learn what you will need to be able to prepare them at home. It is a very simple process, but just like with anything else, it will always goes smoother when you plan ahead.

Because you intend to create these great essential oils to treat headaches and migraines specifically, does this mean that you need to grow some herbs and extract the oils out of them? You surely can. There are 2 different processes used to extract the oils from plants and herbs. You will find below explanations for both methods.

Distillation

In order to use this technique, you will have to equip yourself with a distillation kit. You can choose from many options. These kits come with stainless steel copper or iron distillers. The pricing can vary from anywhere $125 USD up to several thousands of dollars. But usually, for about $200 USD you can purchase a perfectly acceptable distillation kit and start making these essential oils at home. You can find a step by step guide usually with the kit you purchase, but we will briefly summarize the distillation process for you below.

Steam distillation is probably the most well-known technique for essential oil extraction from plants. The essential oils need to come from special parts of the plant, called glands. Steam distillation is a very efficient process for collecting these glands. The distillation requires separating some of the components of the plants while heating. During the process, small sacs of essential oils burst and carry the oil out of the chamber and into a chilled condenser. At that point, the oil and water get separated, and the oil gets impregnated by the herbs and plant scent. The quality of the oil will depend on the temperature and pressure used throughout the process. Watch out for too high a temperate, or the oil could get altered and this would not be good. Allow the extraction process to complete, in order of the oil components from the plant to be released.

Infusion

People use different oils for infusion and it is certainly a personal choice. However, it is better to use an oil that does not have a strong smell to avoid overpowering the herbs' scent. For example, the grapeseed oil is a good one, it is light and has a thin consistency. It has a nice greenish color but hardly any scent. Almond oil is also a great one to use as well, and exudes a sweet nutty smell and is rich in vitamin E and oleic acid. Let the plants and flowers take over the essential oil created. You can also select any other vegetable oil such as olive or coconut oil. Although the olive oil might have a stronger scent, it is very easy to find in a store. The coconut oil is solid at room temperature and offers a long life shelf. Shea butter is another option and also solid at room temperature. You simply have to select the oil or oil mix you prefer with which to make your own special essential oils.

What is great about this process is that you really do not need any specialized equipment, so it can be done with what you already own. You will need the following:

- the oil of your choice

- herbs, flowers, plants to be infused

- clean glass jars

- coffee filters or cheesecloth's

- funnel

- spoon

- pan or skillet

Simple infused method

It is recommended to sterilize the glass jars and bottles you will use to store your essential oils by running them through the dishwasher. Next, you need to prepare the herbs you will be working with by thoroughly washing and drying the fresh herbs. Then place them in the clean jars.

Add the oil of your choice, making sure it completely covers the herbs before closing the lid. You will need to have a sunny spot for which to place your jars. You will leave the jar alone for about a week, making sure you shake it gently every day.

Next it will be time to strain. You can taste the oil to make sure it has the desired flavor, and if it needs to infuse longer, simply close the lid and wait another 3 or 4 days. If it is ready, drain the oil into a new clean jar, using a coffee filter or cheesecloth. Then make sure to store it in a cool place or in the refrigerator.

Heating method

This method will requires the same equipment, and it is actually an accelerated way to infuse the herbs by using heat.

Heat up the oil and the spices or herbs in a skillet until you see the oil bubbling—no longer than 5 minutes should be required. Strain into a clean jar and let it cool down. When it is cool enough, place the lid on, and store appropriately.

You can also use the heat differently and decide to heat up the jar all together. This mean that you will place the herbs in a clean jar and cover them with oil as previously instructed. Then you simply place the jar on a heating plate and let it overpower your house with that wonderful smell for about 3 hours. When the flavor seems right to you, drain the herbs with a cheesecloth or coffee filter, poor and store once cooled down in a clean jar.

Chapter 3: Essential Oils Recipes To Treat Migraines And Headaches

Now, it's time to get to the heart of this book and explain what herbs you should use to treat migraines and headaches. You might have to try a few of them to find the perfect combination of herbs to help soothe these debilitating attacks of head pain. Don't feel like you have failed if you don't succeed the first time, just like a chef has to try mixing in ingredients several times before creating the perfect recipe, you might need a few tries to get it right.

Bergamot

- Bergamot is used to treat stress, anxiety, depression, skin infections, fatigue, and is also effective at treating headaches.

- Bergamot has a delightful light citrus scent. (it is a cross between an orange and lemon). This fruit's oil however contain an ingredient that can become toxic if exposed to sunlight. So, be careful and keep your bottles in a cool dark place.

- To treat headaches or other sources of pain, use a drop of Bergamot oil with a few teaspoons of coconut or avocado oil and rub it on your skin, where you are experiencing the pain. This oil will help by releasing some hormones into your body causing you to be less sensitive to pain.

- You can also use this oil in a diffuser safely. It is however not recommended to take it orally unless advised and supervised by an expert.

Chamomile

- It is good to know that chamomile can also help you reduce inflammation and fight bacteria because of its multiple beneficial properties.

- The flowers of this plant can also, of course, relieve pain form headaches and migraines. The analgesic properties of the plant can not only help your head pain, but can relieve muscle and joint pain, sinuses, toothaches and bone injuries.

- Also, it acts as an antispasmodic, meaning it can help in reducing nervous system issues.

- To use this fantastic oil, you can simply drop a few drops into your favorite herbal tea. You can also decide to diffuse the oil at home before bedtime or when you are experiencing headaches or migraines.

- You could also mix chamomile, lavender oils (10 drops of each) and wild orange oil (5 drops), in a small spray bottle. Before your nap or while resting form a headache, spray on your comforter or pillows.

Clary Sage

- Clary sage oil can greatly help women because of its hormone-like components. It can help in soothing menopausal issues (hot flashes), menstrual pain, and can even help reduce muscle pain. Clary sage can definitely help regulate blood pressure and treat fatigue as well as some respiratory illnesses.

- Clary sage can also help with our main focus— reducing headaches and migraines. It can additionally help improve memory, reduce anxiety and stimulate mental activity.

- You can use the sage oil just like the lavender oil, and add a few drops into your warm bath to ease your pain due to headaches.

- You can directly rub the oil behind your neck and that stiffness and pain will amazingly go away pretty fast.

- Use it in your diffuser, along with peppermint and/or orange, you will love the smell and feel the benefits. If you use it before bedtime, it will also help you relax as well.

Eucalyptus

- Eucalyptus can also be used to fight migraines, but also fevers, respiratory issues (inflammation), and bacterial infections, so let's see how it can relieve this awful pain we often experience.

- Because Eucalyptus works as an expectorant, it will help in opening your nasal passageways and reduce that sinus pressure that is often responsible for these terrible headaches.

- Dilute two or three drops of eucalyptus oil with a carrier oil, and massage it on your chest, back of your neck, temples, and forehead. It will actively work on eliminating the nasal congestion and relieve that tension to liberate you from headaches, or even from migraines.

- Also, use eucalyptus oil to kill the mold in your house instead of bleach. This will greatly assist with any symptoms of headaches associated with allergies or the presence of mold.

Jasmine

- The flower of the plant is used to help make this essential oil. It can be used for many purposes such as a sleeping aid and sedative.

- So, not only will jasmine help you get relief when you have headaches but it will also relieve anxiety, stress and many mood disorders such as depression. It can help with inflammation in your body as well.

- Apply the jasmine oil on your pulse points and soothe your nervous tension or place a dab of oil in your hands, rub them together and inhale deeply for relief.

Ginger root

- I am sure you already know the numerous benefits of ginger when you use it in cooking. Now, learn how to use the ginger root to get rid of headaches and migraines.

- Ginger oil can also help with many other health conditions such as digestion, inflammation, heart conditions, respiratory problems and menstrual disorders. It even has some aphrodisiac properties!

- Rub two or three drops of the essential oil on your forehead, temples and beck and wait for sweet relief.

Lavender

- Although lavender is used for many purposes, such as relieving stress, treating depression, as a decongestant, and also as an anti-inflammatory, it can also greatly help with your unpleasant migraines and headaches.

- The reason why lavender can also help reduce headaches lies in the fact that the use of lavender oil will affect your limbic system. So, the linalool included in the lavender is absorbed quickly by the body and can directly play on the nervous system.

- While headaches can be reduced, other conditions can also be prevented, that could potentially be the cause of headaches. Lavender oil will help reduce feelings of restlessness and agitated sleep. Because it regulates the serotinin levels well, it can also help minimize the pain in the nervous system synonymous with potential migraines.

- In order to use the lavender oil efficiently, you can apply a few drops of the lavender oil directly on the back of your neck, temples and wrists, and this should help in relieving headache symptoms.

- Another way to use lavender oil, is to add it into your warm bath. Use approximately 10 drops in your warm bath water and take long deep breathes while bathing to maximize the tension relieving properties of the lavender oil.

- Finally you can also use a drop of lavender oil at home or in your office, to help reduce stress muscle tension and help boosting your moral, your mood

Lemongrass

- Lemongrass oil offers many benefits such as headache relief, energy boost, germ killing agent, muscle pain reliever, stomach pain soother and fever reducer. But again, let's concentrate on how to reduce headaches.

- Create your own lemongrass body scrub. Combine 10 drops of lemongrass, coconut oil and Epsom salt. While showering, apply everywhere, including your temples, forehead neck and shoulders to help relieve pain.

- You can actually use the lemongrass oil "au natural" and rub it where you need some pain relief. Also, use the diffuser to create a calm atmosphere before bedtime as lemongrass oil is known to relieve anxiety, irritability and help fight insomnia.

Oregano

- Although oregano has been mainly used in the past to treat symptoms of cold and flu as well as bloating, earaches and fatigue, it appears that it can also be efficient in helping reduce migraines and headaches.

- You can actually ingest it directly. Use three drops of oregano oil under the tongue, at the first sign of a migraine or headache and see how you feel. Beware of the very strong taste, it will surprise you, but it is harmless.

- Oregano seems to also have anti-inflammatory properties and you can find it in capsule form at your drugstore if you don't like taking the oil orally.

- Because it such a great decongestant, if you are experimenting headaches due to congestion, oregano oil can make a difference. Try to use a mixture of oregano oil and olive oil (50/50), and run between your eyebrows, your forehead and temples. Be careful, do not get it in your eyes.

Peppermint

- You can actually apply peppermint oil directly on your forehead and temples to relieve headaches.

- It is also recommended to use a combination of peppermint oil, eucalyptus oil and ethanol (alcohol) to treat head discomfort. Do not use regular rubbing alcohol, but instead look for grain alcohol. When peppermint is mixed with ethanol is usually helps reducing sensitivity while experiencing headaches.

- Another great way to use peppermint oil is to dilute it with two or three drops of coconut oil. Use a cotton ball and rub this mixture on your neck, shoulders and forehead, right next to your hairline. Reapply 2 or 3 times. You should feel better in about 30 minutes after applying. If you have not experienced relief within an hour, reapply the essential oil. Peppermint oils are not recommended for small children.

- You can make your own mix using one of the suggested methods in the previous chapter or you can find peppermint oil in pharmacy or natural food stores.

- On top of relieving your headaches, Peppermint can help sharpen your focus, enhance your mental alertness, and act as an energy booster.

Rosemary

- Rosemary oil can also help relieve symptoms associated with headaches. In fact it will help reduce stress or emotional triggers, by giving its user some great calming benefits.

- Additionally, Rosemary can help in relieving inflammation, blood circulation problems, upset stomachs and digestion problems.

- Use one drop of rosemary oil in your tea, water or soup and you can help soothe your migraine.

- Also, to help relieve frequent headaches rub your temples, back of the neck and forehead a few drops of rosemary oil mixed with either peppermint or coconut oil.

Sandalwood

- Sandalwood oil is extracted directly from the trees mainly found in Indian territories.

- The oil offers many properties, such as mental clarity, alertness, and calming and relaxing effect. It is also known to act as a memory booster and help in fighting spasms (nerves, muscles and blood vessels)

- Try using the sandalwood oil in a lamp, to help you get rid of your headache when it occurs. It will certainly at least help you get rid of some of the stress you may be experiencing.

Sweet Marjoram

- This herb has some sedative properties and will definitely help people get relief from spams, stiffness, rheumatisms, insomnia, fatigue, joint pain, stress, colds, asthma, and the even the infamous migraines.

- Note that the marjoram essential oil can blend nicely with chamomile, lemongrass, rosemary, eucalyptus, or even bergamot oils.

- Dilute a few drops and apply in the proper areas, neck, shoulders, and temples to relieve headaches or migraines.

- Also, before bedtime to favor relaxation, use the diffuser with marjoram essential oil.

Thyme

- This herb is certainly widely used in cooking, and now can be used as an essential to treat joints, muscle pain and backache as well as headaches and migraines.

- Use one or two drops of essential thyme oil, or a mix of rosemary oil and thyme oil, and apply on your temples and forehead. Gently rub for a few minutes. It is reportedly almost as efficient as ibuprofen.

- You can also use the thyme essential oil by diluting the oil in fraction of coconut oil and rubbing on the painful areas. Apparently, if you or someone you love have problems with snoring, apply one drop on the big toe before bedtime on a daily basis.

Chapter 4: Additional Tips And FAQ's

Can an essential oil cause a rash or burn on your skin?

Of course it can. Just like any other new substance you would ingest or use against your skin, you can develop some reaction to it. It does not mean you are allergic to it, but it can mean that your skin will get irritated each time it is in contact with that particular essential oil. Some people attribute these reactions to the detoxification process. It is not true. When you are detoxing your body, the process implies you are taking away something, not adding something. So the theory is actually not founded. If your skin develops a rash, or adverse reaction, it is not a good sign, and your body is telling you loud and clear: "*stop what you are doing right now!*" That's why, just like foods, you should always try one essential oil at a time, to make sure you are not developing any kind of reactions and can move on to the next one safely.

Can essential oils expire?

That seems like an important detail. Let's see what science has to say. It is clear that essential oils can degrade with time. Because essential oils are complex mixtures, they are made of many different components. For example, one of them is a carbon atom, such as alcohol, acid or aldehyde. So when one of these ingredients are exposed to air, they will follow the oxidation process. It can be compared to wine that has been stored for too long, turning into vinegar. It is a chemical process and yes inevitably if the essential oil is stored for too long it can expire. So, because of this, it is recommended that you label the essential oil not only with their name but their date of conception.

There are many factors influencing the shelf life of your essentials oils including: the method and conditions of distillation (preparation), the quality of oils, and the storage conditions. However, as a general rule, you can expect your essential oil to last about 1 year from the date of conception. If you want to ensure to keep it as long as possible, bottle it in a darker and smaller bottle. Make sure it is stored in a cool place, or better yet in the refrigerator. To detect if the essential oil is still good or not, examine its consistency, it should not have thickened too much or should not be cloudy looking. Also the aroma needs to be nice and normal, and if it has changed drastically, throw it away.

Can essential oil cure cancer?

Wouldn't' that be wonderful? Many have claimed that essential oils could cure Ebola or even cancer. There has been research going for many years possibly linking frankincense's to cancer prevention. It is a reality that this plant will help support better immune systems, and fight infections.

In 2013, a study conducted at the University of Leicester England, arrived at the conclusion that a compound included in frankincense can help with preventing or treating certain cancer cells such as breast, colon, stomach, pancreatic or prostate.

No matter where the truth lies at this time. Many cancer patients have found some type of relief using aromatherapy. They use essential oils mainly to relieve certain symptoms due to chemotherapy or even some cancer symptoms they might experience. It is easy to buy a home diffuser and some oils and use aromatherapy to relief some the pain due to cancer, but not everyone will react the same way or benefit from essential oils the same way.

Can essential oils really replace certain prescription drugs all together?

There is a lot of talk about the benefits of essential oils and how they could efficiently replace certain antibiotics. For example, many people use the oil of oregano to treat minor infections, runny nose, ear ache, achiness, and sore throat. The antiseptic power of certain oils, such as thyme, clove, cinnamon, peppermint, lemongrass, mint, and rosemary can help with many cold symptoms and, to a certain extent, replace antibiotics if the symptoms improve in a timely matter. Essentials oils also have many antimicrobial, antibacterial, and antifungal properties, and always have. So to think that they can be an alternative to antibiotics, is not far off. Essential oils have been used on humans for thousands of years, but now it seems like the pharmaceutical industries have taken over and to prove to the public the true benefits of the use of essential oils can be a challenging endeavor.

It is very important to be cautious and to consult with your primary care physician or pharmacist with any doubts or questions. You obviously should not get off certain medications for chronic conditions, such as diabetes or high blood pressure, and start using essential oils. Yes, there could be an alternative treatment, but you want to do it safely, and certainly under the supervision of a health care professional.

Special Bonus

To thank you for purchasing my guide, I have specifically prepared the bonus "**Aromatherapy – First Aid Kit**" report for you. This report will show you how you can heal yourself inside out using the power of aromatherapy

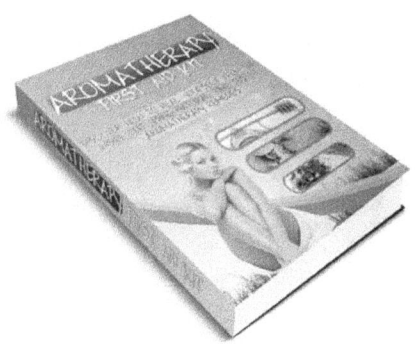

Inside this report, you will find:

1. Secrets to a natural beauty and great looking skin

2. How you can make your own perfumes and hair care treatment

3. And many more….

To download this special bonus, simply visit this URL below:

http://giveaway.kindleheaven.com/index.php/essential-oils-aromatherapy/

….And put in both your name and email there so I know who to address and which email address to send the report to.

Conclusion

So next time you experience a headache, or worse, a migraine, please try to use essential oils to relief these unpleasant symptoms. Better yet, try to prevent these headaches by using the essential oils on a regular basis to help you relax. Many essential oils made from herbs and plants can help you sleep better and breathe better, so you can sometimes chase away any headaches before they land. Also, these oils can often help you fight infections, colds, and sinus congestion that will eventually give you a very bad headache.

Now that you know how easily you can make your own essential oils, there is no reason for you to have to run to the pharmacy at the last minute trying to find the right medicine to treat your headache. Always keep one or two essential oils that will relieve any pain in your house, and maybe one at work as well. Make sure you label them, and keep them in a dark and cool storage area. Learn how to mix certain essential oils to change it up and even increase theeir efficiency at times.

Whether you decide to use the herbs you have grown in your own garden or the ones you buy at the fresh market, it does not matter. What matters is that you do use a good infusing or distillation oil, such as the grapeseed oil, for example. Respect the principles for each technique, and always smell and taste the oils once you think they are done, before bottling them, in case they need to remain infusing for a longer period.

Essential oils have been around for a long time. You might just have started using them, and that's ok, because it's never too late to make some healthy changes in your life. They will help you treat many health conditions, including inflammation, respiratory problems, stress, anxiety, sleep problems, mood disorders, digestive and stomach issues, skin problems and can even contribute in your life as an aphrodisiac.

Educate yourself. Read about their use, and regroup with friends to make them on a Saturday afternoon. You could make several batches for even cheaper and make this process even more fun than it already is. If you are uncertain of their interaction with certain medications you are currently taking, please consult with a pharmacist, a natural foods specialist or your pharmacy or doctor for additional advice.

Most of all, most essential oils are not made to take orally, you can usually rub them on your body without danger. To make sure you do not have any allergic reactions, always test on a very small of your body (your hand), for example, before applying anywhere else.

-- Jeanne Hill

www.ingramcontent.com/pod-product-compliance
Lightning Source LLC
Chambersburg PA
CBHW072028280526
45788CB00007B/2719